# NUTRIBULLET SUPERFOOD SMOOTHIES
## 100 MOUTHWATERING, ULTRA-HEALTHY, & SUPER FILLING SMOOTHIE RECIPES

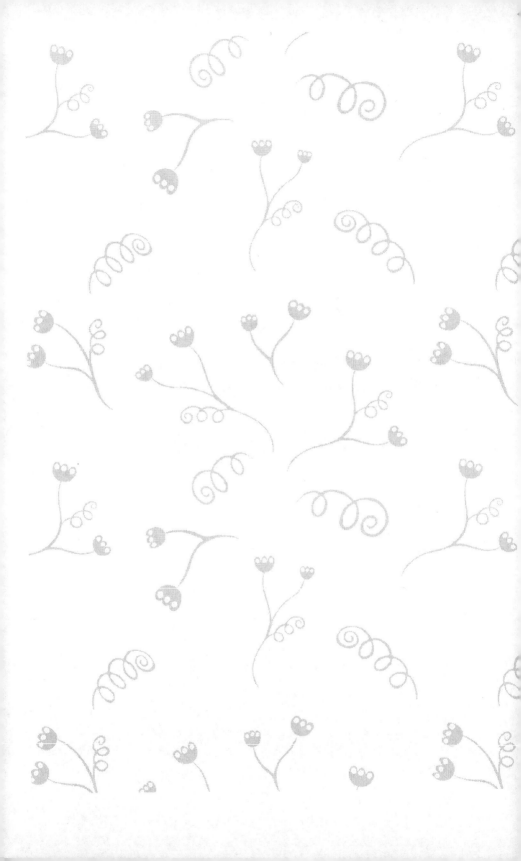

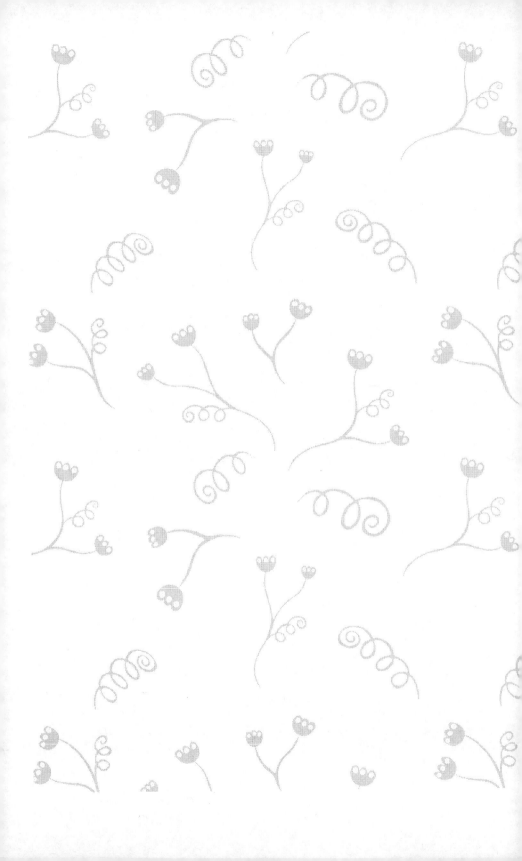

# TABLE OF CONTENTS

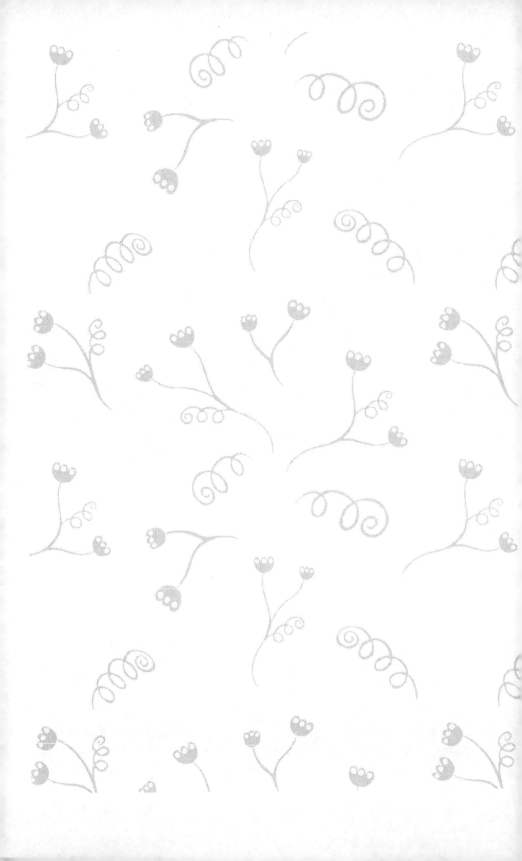

# INTRODUCTION

So you've discovered the awesome power of a NutriBullet? Congratulations.

Suddenly you have a secret weapon: the ability to turn not-exactly-mouthwatering foods like broccoli, kale, spinach, and flaxseed into delicious smoothies that you actually enjoy!

But maybe you're suffering from NutriBullet-itis. You know, the tendency to throw a bunch of healthy foods willy-nilly into the blender and hope for the best. Or maybe you're just eating the same 4 or 5 foods over and over again.

NutriBullet Superfood Smoothies take your NutriBullet smoothies to a new level. More superfoods, more delicious, more filling!

This recipe book provides all the recipes you need to embark on your journey to a healthier, yummier, more energetic lifestyle, one smoothie at a time.

So get out your NutriBullet and let's go!

3

# SWEET-TALKIN' PINEAPPLE CHILL

INGREDIENTS:
¾ CUP GREEN GRAPES
2 TABLESPOONS FLAXSEED
½ GREEN APPLE
½ CUP PINEAPPLE
1 CUP ICE
1 CUP WATER

210 CALORIES

Low in saturated fat
No cholesterol
Very low in sodium
High in dietary fiber
High in iron
Very high in manganese
High in thiamin
Very high in vitamin B6
Very high in vitamin C

# MINTY GREEN GOBLIN

INGREDIENTS:
2 ½ CUPS FRESH BABY SPINACH
1 HANDFUL FRESH MINT LEAVES
2 MEDIUM PEARS
1 TABLESPOON LIME JUICE
1 GREEN APPLE
1 CUP ICE
1 CUP WATER

## 315 CALORIES

Very low in saturated fat
No cholesterol
Low in sodium
Very high in dietary fiber
High in manganese
Very high in vitamin A
Very high in vitamin B6
Very high in vitamin C

# COCO-NUTTY CRUSH

INGREDIENTS:
1 ½ CUPS BABY SPINACH
½ CUP VANILLA YOGURT
½ MEDIUM APPLE
½ CUP COCONUT
1 CUP ICE
1 CUP WATER

425 CALORIES

Very low in cholesterol
High in dietary fiber
High in vitamin A
Very high in vitamin B6

6

# TROPICAL TITAN

INGREDIENTS:
1 CUP KALE
½ CUP PINEAPPLE
½ CUP MANGO CHUNKS
1 FROZEN BANANA
½ CUP VANILLA YOGURT
1 CUP ICE
1 CUP UNSWEETENED COCONUT ALMOND MILK BLEND

## 380 CALORIES

Low in cholesterol
Very high in calcium
Very high in manganese
High in phosphorus
High in potassium
Very high in vitamin A
Very high in vitamin C
Very high in vitamin E

# MR. MELON

INGREDIENTS:
1 CUP CANTALOUPE
1 CUP HONEYDEW MELON
1 CUP ROMAINE LETTUCE
1 TABLESPOON CHIA SEED
1 CUP ICE
1 CUP WATER

180 CALORIES

Very low in saturated fat
No cholesterol
Low in sodium
High in dietary fiber
High in magnesium
High in potassium
Very high in vitamin A
Very high in vitamin B6
Very high in vitamin C

# PICK-ME-UP PEAR

INGREDIENTS:
2 PEARS
2 CUPS FRESH BABY SPINACH
1 FROZEN BANANA
1 CUP ICE
1 CUP WATER

315 CALORIES

Very low in saturated fat
No cholesterol
Very low in sodium
Very high in dietary fiber
Very high in vitamin A
Very high in vitamin C

# CRAZY CUCUMBER-APPLE

INGREDIENTS:
2 CUCUMBERS
1 APPLE
1 CUP ICE
1 CUP UNSWEETENED ALMOND MILK

## 215 CALORIES

Low in saturated fat
No cholesterol
Very high in calcium
High in dietary fiber
High in manganese
High in potassium
High in vitamin A
Very high in vitamin B6
Very high in vitamin C
Very high in vitamin E

# NEW ZEALAND PUNCH

INGREDIENTS:
2 KIWIS
1 CUCUMBER
1 CUP FROZEN BROCCOLI
1 GREEN APPLE
1 TABLESPOON CHIA SEED
1 CUP ICE
1 CUP WATER

## 325 CALORIES

Very low in saturated fat
No cholesterol
Very low in sodium
Very high in dietary fiber
High in potassium
Very high in vitamin B6
Very high in vitamin C

# AGE-DEFYING AVOCADO

**INGREDIENTS:**
½ AVOCADO, PITTED AND PEELED
1 CUP HONEYDEW MELON
½ CUP FROZEN BLUEBERRIES
1 CUP ICE
1 CUP UNSWEETENED COCONUT ALMOND MILK BLEND

**350 CALORIES**

No cholesterol
Low in sodium
High in calcium
High in dietary fiber
Very high in vitamin B6
Very high in vitamin C
High in vitamin E

# CANDY LION DETOX

INGREDIENTS:
3 CUPS DANDELION GREENS
1 BANANA
1 CUP STRAWBERRIES
½ CUP BLUEBERRIES
1 CUP ICE
1 CUP WATER

260 CALORIES

Low in saturated fat
No cholesterol
Low in sodium
High in calcium
High in dietary fiber
High in iron
Very high in manganese
High in magnesium
High in potassium
High in riboflavin
Very high in vitamin A
Very high in vitamin B6
Very high in vitamin C

# BOK CHOY BANG!

**INGREDIENTS:**
1 ½ CUPS FRESH PINEAPPLE
1 MEDIUM HEAD BOK CHOY
1 CUP BABY SPINACH
1 LARGE CUCUMBER
1 APPLE
1 CUP ICE
1 CUP WATER

**275 CALORIES**

Very low in saturated fat
No cholesterol
High in calcium
High in dietary fiber
High in iron
Very high in manganese
High in magnesium
Very high in potassium
High in riboflavin
High in thiamin
Very high in vitamin A
Very high in vitamin B6
Very high in vitamin C

# WATERMELON MAMA

INGREDIENTS:
2 CUPS FRESH WATERMELON
1 MEDIUM BUNCH FRESH PARSLEY
1 LARGE PEACH
1 APPLE
½ CUP GREEN GRAPES
1 CUP ICE
1 CUP UNSWEETENED COCONUT ALMOND MILK BLEND

## 350 CALORIES

Low in saturated fat
No cholesterol
Low in sodium
High in calcium
High in dietary fiber
High in vitamin A
Very high in vitamin B6
Very high in vitamin C
High in vitamin E

# GO-GO GOJI

INGREDIENTS:
3 CUPS FRESH BABY SPINACH
1 CUP GOJI BERRIES
2 FROZEN BANANAS, SLICED
1 CUP RASPBERRIES
1 CUP ICE
1 CUP UNSWEETENED COCONUT ALMOND MILK BLEND

430 CALORIES

Low in saturated fat
No cholesterol
High in calcium
High in dietary fiber
Very high in iron
High in manganese
High in potassium
Very high in vitamin A
Very high in vitamin C

# CHERRY BERRY CHILLER

INGREDIENTS:
1 CUP BLACK CHERRIES (PITTED)
1 CUP GREEN GRAPES
½ CUP BLACKBERRIES
1 CUP BABY SPINACH LEAVES
2 CUPS ICE
1 CUP WATER

## 180 CALORIES

Very low in saturated fat
No cholesterol
Low in sodium
High in dietary fiber
Very high in manganese
Very high in vitamin A
Very high in vitamin C

# APPLE IN A PEAR TREE

INGREDIENTS:
2 PEARS
1 APPLE
1 TABLESPOON CHIA SEED
1 CUP BABY SPINACH
1 CUP ICE
1 CUP WATER

320 CALORIES

Very low in saturated fat
No cholesterol
Very low in sodium
Very high in dietary fiber
High in vitamin A
Very high in vitamin B6
High in vitamin C

# LUSCIOUS LIME TWIST

INGREDIENTS:
1 CUP KALE
1 CUP GRAPES
2 CUPS HONEYDEW MELON
1 APPLE
1 SMALL HANDFUL MINT LEAVES
JUICE OF 1 LIME
1 CUP ICE
1 CUP COCONUT WATER

## 370 CALORIES

Very low in saturated fat
No cholesterol
Low in sodium
Very high in manganese
High in potassium
Very high in vitamin A
Very high in vitamin B6
Very high in vitamin C

# SWEET GULA GULA

**INGREDIENTS:**
1 CUP ARUGULA
2 BANANAS
1 CUP PINEAPPLE
1 CUCUMBER
1 CUP ICE
1 CUP WATER

**340 CALORIES**

Very low in saturated fat
No cholesterol
Very low in sodium
High in dietary fiber
Very high in manganese
High in potassium
High in vitamin B6
Very high in vitamin C

# GREEN PEPPER GODDESS

INGREDIENTS:
2 LARGE GREEN PEPPERS
1 CUP GRAPES
1 LARGE CUCUMBER
1 CUP FRESH PINEAPPLE
1 CUP ICE
1 CUP UNSWEETENED ALMOND MILK

## 280 CALORIES

Very low in saturated fat
No cholesterol
High in calcium
High in dietary fiber
Very high in manganese
High in potassium
High in thiamin
High in vitamin A
High in vitamin B6
Very high in vitamin C
High in vitamin E

# THE BIG GREEN MONSTER

INGREDIENTS:
1 CUP BABY SPINACH
1 CUP ROMAINE LETTUCE
1 LARGE CUCUMBER
2 GREEN APPLES
2 KIWIS
1 CUP ICE
1 CUP WATER

## 340 CALORIES

Very low in saturated fat
No cholesterol
Very low in sodium
High in dietary fiber
High in potassium
Very high in vitamin A
Very high in vitamin B6
Very high in vitamin C

# COCO-CARROT CRAZE

INGREDIENTS:
1 CUP ROMAINE LETTUCE
2 LARGE CARROTS
1 CUP HONEYDEW MELON
1 CUP ICE
1 CUP COCONUT WATER
1 CUP COCONUT ALMOND MILK BLEND

## 220 CALORIES

No cholesterol
Very high in calcium
High in dietary fiber
High in manganese
High in potassium
Very high in vitamin A
High in vitamin B6
Very high in vitamin C
Very high in vitamin E

# STRAWBERRY BANANA BONANZA

INGREDIENTS:
1 HEAD OF BOK CHOY
1 BANANA
1 CUP STRAWBERRIES
1 TABLESPOON CHIA SEEDS
1 CUP ICE
1 CUP WATER

320 CALORIES

Very low in saturated fat
No cholesterol
Very high in calcium
Very high in dietary fiber
High in iron
Very high in manganese
High in magnesium
High in phosphorus
Very high in potassium
High in riboflavin
Very high in vitamin A
Very high in vitamin B6
Very high in vitamin C

# PAPAYA MANGO MADNESS

INGREDIENTS:
1 PAPAYA, PEELED AND SEEDS REMOVED
1 CUP MANGO CHUNKS
1 CUP PINEAPPLE
2 CUPS BABY SPINACH
1 CUP ICE
1 CUP UNSWEETENED COCONUT ALMOND MILK BLEND

410 CALORIES

Low in saturated fat
No cholesterol
Low in sodium
High in calcium
High in dietary fiber
Very high in manganese
Very high in vitamin A
Very high in vitamin C
High in vitamin E

# POMEGRANATE CELERY SPLASH

INGREDIENTS:
2 CUPS FRESH BABY SPINACH
1 CUP POMEGRANATE JUICE
4 CELERY STALKS
1 FUJI APPLE
1 CUP ICE
1 CUP WATER

270 CALORIES

Very low in saturated fat
No cholesterol
Low in sodium
High in potassium
Very high in vitamin A
Very high in vitamin B6
Very high in vitamin C

# RAD RASPBERRY TWIST

INGREDIENTS:
1 CUP POMEGRANATE JUICE
1 CUP FRESH BABY SPINACH
1 CUP ROMAINE LETTUCE
2 CUPS RED RASPBERRIES
1 CUP ICE
1 CUP WATER

## 285 CALORIES

Very low in saturated fat
No cholesterol
Very low in sodium
High in dietary fiber
Very high in vitamin A
Very high in vitamin C

# RASPBERRY WATER COOLER

INGREDIENTS:
1 CUP RASPBERRIES
1 CUP FRESH WATERMELON
1 CUP ROMAINE LETTUCE
3 CELERY STALKS
1 APPLE
1 CUP ICE
1 CUP WATER

## 220 CALORIES

Very low in saturated fat
No cholesterol
Low in sodium
Very high in dietary fiber
High in manganese
High in vitamin A
Very high in vitamin B6
Very high in vitamin C

# AWESOME APPLE RAPINI

INGREDIENTS:
2 CUPS RAPINI
2 GREEN APPLES
1 LARGE BANANA
1 CUP ICE
1 CUP WATER

360 CALORIES

Very low in saturated fat
No cholesterol
Very low in sodium
High in dietary fiber
Very high in vitamin A
Very high in vitamin B6
Very high in vitamin C

# BEET GREEN BLAST-OFF

INGREDIENTS:
2 CUPS BEET GREENS
1 GREEN APPLE
2 CUPS GREEN GRAPES
1 LARGE BANANA
1 CUP ICE
1 CUP WATER

350 CALORIES

Very low in saturated fat
No cholesterol
High in dietary fiber
Very high in manganese
High in potassium
Very high in vitamin A
Very high in vitamin B6
Very high in vitamin C

# FIGGY BANANA

**INGREDIENTS:**
**4 LARGE FIGS**
**2 BANANAS**
**2 CUPS BABY SPINACH**
**1 CUP ICE**
**1 CUP WATER**

**410 CALORIES**

Very low in saturated fat
No cholesterol
Very low in sodium
High in dietary fiber
High in manganese
High in potassium
Very high in vitamin A
High in vitamin B6
High in vitamin C

# WATERMELON WAKE-UP

INGREDIENTS:
2 CUPS WATERMELON
1 CUP ROMAINE LETTUCE
3 CELERY STALKS
1 ORANGE
1 HANDFUL FRESH MINT LEAVES
1 CUP ICE
1 CUP WATER

## 200 CALORIES

Very low in saturated fat
No cholesterol
Low in sodium
High in dietary fiber
High in potassium
Very high in vitamin A
High in vitamin B6
Very high in vitamin C

# BANANA BERRY BLIZZARD

INGREDIENTS:
2 FROZEN BANANAS
1 CUP RASPBERRIES
1 CUP STRAWBERRIES
2 CUPS FRESH SPINACH
1 CUP ICE
1 CUP UNSWEETENED ALMOND MILK

## 360 CALORIES

Very low in saturated fat
No cholesterol
High in calcium
Very high in dietary fiber
Very high in manganese
High in magnesium
High in potassium
Very high in vitamin A
High in vitamin B6
Very high in vitamin C
High in vitamin E

# BROCCOLI KIWI BASH

INGREDIENTS:
3 KIWI FRUITS
1 CUP BROCCOLI
1 GREEN APPLE
1 CUP GRAPES
1 CUP ICE
1 CUP UNSWEETENED ALMOND MILK

350 CALORIES

Very low in saturated fat
No cholesterol
High in calcium
High in dietary fiber
High in manganese
High in potassium
Very high in vitamin B6
Very high in vitamin C
High in vitamin E

# MANGO GREEN TEA MADNESS

INGREDIENTS:
1 CUP FRESH BABY SPINACH
1 CUP ROMAINE LETTUCE
1 ½ CUPS PINEAPPLE
1 MANGO, PEELED AND DESEEDED
1 BANANA
1 CUP ICE
1 CUP GREEN TEA, BREWED

## 390 CALORIES

Very low in saturated fat
No cholesterol
Very low in sodium
High in dietary fiber
Very high in manganese
Very high in vitamin A
High in vitamin B6
Very high in vitamin C

# THE PERKY PEAR

INGREDIENTS:
1 CUCUMBER
2 PEARS
1 APPLE
1 HANDFUL FRESH MINT LEAVES
1 CUP ICE
1 CUP WATER

340 CALORIES

Very low in saturated fat
No cholesterol
Very low in sodium
High in dietary fiber
Very high in vitamin B6
High in vitamin C

# ADVENTUROUS APRICOT

INGREDIENTS:
6 APRICOTS, DESEEDED
1 CUP KALE
2 APPLES
1 LARGE BANANA
1 CUP ICE
1 CUP WATER

440 CALORIES

Very low in saturated fat
No cholesterol
Very low in sodium
High in dietary fiber
High in manganese
High in potassium
Very high in vitamin A
Very high in vitamin B6
Very high in vitamin C

# BERRY BERRY LOW-CALORIE

INGREDIENTS:
1 CUP FRESH SPINACH
2 CUPS FRESH FROZEN STRAWBERRIES
2 STALKS CELERY
½ CUP RED RASPBERRIES
1 CUP ICE
1 CUP WATER

135 CALORIES

Very low in saturated fat
No cholesterol
Low in sodium
Very high in dietary fiber
High in iron
Very high in manganese
High in magnesium
High in potassium
Very high in vitamin A
Very high in vitamin C

# KOMBUCHA KRAZE

INGREDIENTS:
2 CUPS ROMAINE LETTUCE
½ AVOCADO
2 LARGE FROZEN BANANAS
1 CUP ICE
1 CUP WATER
1 CUP KOMBUCHA TEA

460 CALORIES

No cholesterol
Very low in sodium
High in dietary fiber
Very high in vitamin B6
High in vitamin C

# LUSCIOUS LYCHEE

INGREDIENTS:
15 PIECES LYCHEE FRUITS, PEELED AND DESEEDED
1 CUP SPINACH
1 CUP RADISH GREENS
1 CUP FRESH PINEAPPLE
1 CUP ICE
1 CUP WATER

190 CALORIES

Very low in saturated fat
No cholesterol
Low in sodium
Very high in manganese
Very high in vitamin A
Very high in vitamin C

# MOUTHWATERING MANGO

**INGREDIENTS:**
**2 CUPS FRESH SPINACH**
**2 MANGOES, PEELED AND DESEEDED**
**1 BANANA**
**½ CUP PINEAPPLE**
**1 CUP UNSWEETENED COCONUT ALMOND MILK BLEND**

**350 CALORIES**

Low in saturated fat
No cholesterol
Low in sodium
High in calcium
High in dietary fiber
Very high in manganese
High in potassium
Very high in vitamin A
High in vitamin B6
Very high in vitamin C
High in vitamin E

# RAISIN ROCKER

INGREDIENTS:
2 CUPS RAPINI
1/2 CUP RAISINS
1 BANANA
1 TABLESPOON CHIA SEED
1 CUP ICE
1 CUP WATER

430 CALORIES

Very low in saturated fat
No cholesterol
Very low in sodium
Very high in vitamin A
Very high in vitamin C

# SUCCULENT SWISS CHARD

INGREDIENTS:
2 CUPS SWISS CHARD
2 BANANAS
1 CUP BLUEBERRIES
1 CUP RASPBERRIES
1 CUP ICE
1 CUP WATER

## 371 CALORIES

Very low in saturated fat
No cholesterol
Low in sodium
Very high in dietary fiber
Very high in manganese
High in magnesium
High in potassium
Very high in vitamin A
Very high in vitamin B6
Very high in vitamin C

# COCONUT MELON MIXER

INGREDIENTS:
2 CUPS HONEYDEW MELON
1 CUP FRESH BABY SPINACH
1 CUP ICE
1 CUP COCONUT WATER

## 190 CALORIES

Very low in saturated fat
No cholesterol
High in magnesium
Very high in potassium
Very high in vitamin A
Very high in vitamin C

# BOK CHOY BLISS

INGREDIENTS:
1 CUP RASPBERRIES
2 BANANAS
1 CUP PINEAPPLE
1 CUP BOK CHOY
1 CUP ICE
1 CUP WATER

## 365 CALORIES

Very low in saturated fat
No cholesterol
Very low in sodium
High in dietary fiber
Very high in manganese
High in potassium
High in vitamin A
High in vitamin B6
Very high in vitamin C

# TROPICAL COCONUT COOLER

INGREDIENTS:
1 CUP PINEAPPLE
1/4 CUP UNSWEETENED COCONUT FLAKES
1 BANANA
1 MANGO, PEELED AND DESEEDED
2 APRICOTS, DESEEDED
2 CUPS FRESH BABY SPINACH
1 CUP ICE
1 CUP WATER

480 CALORIES

No cholesterol
Very low in sodium
High in dietary fiber
Very high in manganese
Very high in vitamin A
Very high in vitamin C

# EXOTIC ELDERBERRY

## INGREDIENTS:
1 CUP ELDERBERRIES
1 CUP SWISS CHARD
2 BANANAS
1 CUP ICE
1 CUP WATER

## 320 CALORIES

Very low in saturated fat
No cholesterol
Low in sodium
Very high in dietary fiber
High in manganese
High in potassium
High in vitamin A
High in vitamin B6
Very high in vitamin C

# TRIPLE BERRYLICIOUS

INGREDIENTS:
1 CUP STRAWBERRIES
1 CUP BLACKBERRIES
1 CUP RASPBERRIES
1 CUP FRESH BABY SPINACH
2 TABLESPOONS FLAXSEED
½ CUP VANILLA YOGURT
1 CUP ICE
1 CUP WATER

340 CALORIES

Very low in cholesterol
Low in sodium
High in calcium
Very high in dietary fiber
High in iron
Very high in manganese
High in magnesium
High in phosphorus
High in vitamin A
Very high in vitamin B6
Very high in vitamin C

# FAB FRUIT COCKTAIL

INGREDIENTS:
1 PEAR
½ CUP CHERRIES, DESEEDED
½ CUP PEACHES
1 CUP RAPINI
1 CUP ICE
1 CUP WATER

140 CALORIES

Very low in saturated fat
No cholesterol
Low in sodium
High in dietary fiber
Very high in vitamin A
Very high in vitamin C

# CUCUMBER PEAR PIZAZZ

INGREDIENTS:
1 PEAR
1 CUCUMBER
4 STALKS CELERY
1 CUP TURNIP GREENS
1 APPLE
½ CUP VANILLA YOGURT
1 CUP ICE
1 CUP WATER

330 CALORIES

Low in saturated fat
Very low in cholesterol
High in calcium
High in dietary fiber
High in potassium
Very high in vitamin A
Very high in vitamin B6
Very high in vitamin C

# CHERRY PARSLEY PUNCH

INGREDIENTS:
1 HANDFUL FRESH PARSLEY
1 HEAD ROMAINE LETTUCE
2 CUPS BLACK CHERRIES, PITTED
1 APPLE
1 CUP ICE
1 CUP WATER

## 400 CALORIES

No saturated fat
No cholesterol
Low in sodium
High in dietary fiber
High in iron
Very high in vitamin B6
High in vitamin C

# DRAGON FRUIT DASH

INGREDIENTS:
1 LARGE DRAGON FRUIT
2 FROZEN BANANAS
1 HEAD OF BOK CHOY
1 CUP ICE
1 CUP WATER

## 360 CALORIES

Very low in saturated fat
No cholesterol
Very high in calcium
High in dietary fiber
High in iron
Very high in manganese
High in magnesium
Very high in potassium
High in riboflavin
Very high in vitamin A
Very high in vitamin B6
Very high in vitamin C

# GREEN TEA GEISHA

INGREDIENTS:
2 CUPS KALE
1 PEAR
2 CUPS CUBED MANGO
2 CELERY STALKS
1 CUP ICE
BREWED GREEN TEA

300 CALORIES

Very low in saturated fat
No cholesterol
Low in sodium
High in dietary fiber
High in manganese
High in potassium
Very high in vitamin A
High in vitamin B6
Very high in vitamin C

# MANGO ISLAND ICE

INGREDIENTS:
¼ CUP UNSWEETENED COCONUT FLAKES
2 MANGOES, PEELED AND DESEEDED
JUICE OF 1 LIME
1 CUP PINEAPPLE
1 CUP KALE
1 CUP ICE
1 CUP ALMOND MILK COCONUT MILK BLEND

## 450 CALORIES

No cholesterol
Low in sodium
High in calcium
Very high in manganese
Very high in vitamin A
Very high in vitamin C
High in vitamin E

# KICKIN' KEFIR

INGREDIENTS:
½ CUP ALFALFA SPROUTS
1 CUP LOW-FAT VANILLA KEFIR
1 CUP BABY SPINACH
JUICE OF 1 LIME
2 CUPS FRESH PINEAPPLE
1 CUP ICE
1 CUP WATER

350 CALORIES

Low in saturated fat
Low in cholesterol
Low in sodium
High in calcium
Very high in manganese
Very high in vitamin A
Very high in vitamin C

# SPIRULINA SPLASH

INGREDIENTS:
1 CUP ROMAINE LETTUCE
2 ORANGES, PEELED
½ CUP STRAWBERRIES
2 TBSP. SPIRULINA POWDER
1 CUP PLAIN YOGURT
1 CUP ICE
1 CUP WATER

## 420 CALORIES

Low in cholesterol
High in calcium
High in dietary fiber
High in phosphorus
High in potassium
High in riboflavin
High in thiamin
High in vitamin B6
Very high in vitamin C

# KIWI-KALE FILLER-UPPER

**INGREDIENTS:**
**1 CUP KALE**
**5 KIWI FRUITS**
**1 TABLESPOON FLAXSEED**
**1 TABLESPOON CHIA SEEDS**
**1 CUP ICE**
**1 CUP WATER**

**360 CALORIES**

Very low in saturated fat
No cholesterol
Very low in sodium
Very high in dietary fiber
High in manganese
High in magnesium
High in potassium
Very high in vitamin A
Very high in vitamin B6
Very high in vitamin C

# PERSIMMON PARADISE

INGREDIENTS:
2 PERSIMMONS
2 CUPS CHOPPED BOK CHOY
2 BANANAS
1 MANGO, PEELED AND DESEEDED
1 CUP ICE
1 CUP WATER

360 CALORIES

Very low in saturated fat
No cholesterol
Low in sodium
High in dietary fiber
High in manganese
High in potassium
Very high in vitamin A
High in vitamin B6
Very high in vitamin C

# CARIBBEAN CUCUMBER

INGREDIENTS:
2 CUCUMBERS
1 CUP BABY SPINACH
1 CUP PINEAPPLE
¼ CUP UNSWEETENED COCONUT FLAKES
1 CUP ICE
1 CUP UNSWEETENED COCONUT ALMOND MILK BLEND

## 400 CALORIES

No cholesterol
Low in sodium
High in calcium
High in dietary fiber
Very high in manganese
High in vitamin A
Very high in vitamin C
High in vitamin E

# BLUEBERRY BOOST

INGREDIENTS:
1 CUP ROMAINE LETTUCE
1 CUP BLUEBERRIES
1 CUP SPINACH
2 GREEN APPLES
1 CUP ICE
1 CUP WATER

290 CALORIES

Very low in saturated fat
No cholesterol
Very low in sodium
High in dietary fiber
High in iron
High in manganese
High in vitamin A
Very high in vitamin B6
Very high in vitamin C

# POMMELO PLUNGE

INGREDIENTS:
1 POMMELO, PEELED
1 CUP ROMAINE LETTUCE
1 CUP PINEAPPLE
1 CUP ICE
1 CUP WATER

140 CALORIES

Very low in saturated fat
No cholesterol
Very low in sodium
High in dietary fiber
Very high in manganese
Very high in vitamin A
Very high in vitamin B6
Very high in vitamin C

# AWESOME ALOE

INGREDIENTS:
1 CUP RAPINI
3 TABLESPOONS ALOE VERA GEL
1 CUP GREEN GRAPES
2 APPLES
3 KIWI FRUIT
1 CUP ICE
1 CUP WATER

## 410 CALORIES

Very low in saturated fat
No cholesterol
Very low in sodium
High in dietary fiber
Very high in vitamin A
Very high in vitamin B6
Very high in vitamin C

# STRAWBERRY SMASH

INGREDIENTS:
1 CUP RADISH GREENS
1 CUP STRAWBERRIES
2 CELERY STALKS
2 KIWI FRUIT
1 CUP ICE
1 CUP WATER

150 CALORIES

Very low in saturated fat
No cholesterol
Low in sodium
High in calcium
Very high in dietary fiber
High in manganese
High in potassium
Very high in vitamin A
Very high in vitamin C

# GO-GO MELON MACHINE

INGREDIENTS:
1 CUP CANTALOUPE
2 MANGOES, PEELED AND DESEEDED
1 CUP VANILLA YOGURT
2 CUPS ROMAINE LETTUCE
1 CUP ICE
1 CUP WATER

380 CALORIES

Low in cholesterol
High in calcium
High in phosphorus
High in potassium
Very high in vitamin A
High in vitamin B6
Very high in vitamin C

# LYCHEE LAGOON

INGREDIENTS:
15 LYCHEE FRUITS
½ CUP STRAWBERRIES
1 CUP BABY SPINACH
1 CUP ICE
1 CUP COCONUT WATER

155 CALORIES

Very low in saturated fat
No cholesterol
High in manganese
High in potassium
Very high in vitamin A
Very high in vitamin C

# DRAGON FRUIT DELIGHT

INGREDIENTS:
2 DRAGON FRUITS
2 BANANAS
1 CUP SPRING MIX GREENS
1 CUP GREEN GRAPES
1 CUP ICE
1 CUP WATER

400 CALORIES

Very low in saturated fat
No cholesterol
Very low in sodium
High in manganese
High in vitamin B6
High in vitamin C

# WATERMELON MANGO TANGO

INGREDIENTS:
1 CUP WATERMELON
1 MANGO, PEELED AND DESEEDED
1 CUP FRESH BABY SPINACH
1 CUP ICE
1 CUP UNSWEETENED ALMOND MILK

150 CALORIES

Very low in saturated fat
No cholesterol
High in dietary fiber
Very high in vitamin A
Very high in vitamin C

# PARSLEY PEACH FIZZ

INGREDIENTS:
1 HANDFUL FRESH PARSLEY
1 CUP BABY SPINACH
3 PEACHES, DESEEDED
1 CUP GRAPES
1 CUP ICE
1 CUP CLUB SODA

215 CALORIES

Very low in saturated fat
No cholesterol
High in dietary fiber
High in manganese
High in potassium
Very high in vitamin A
Very high in vitamin C

# LYCHEE LEMONADE

**INGREDIENTS:**
15 LYCHEE FRUITS
3 TABLESPOONS LEMON JUICE
1 CUP CANTALOUPE
1 CUP ROMAINE LETTUCE
1 CUP ICE
1 CUP WATER

**160 CALORIES**

Low in saturated fat
No cholesterol
Low in sodium
Very high in vitamin A
High in vitamin B6
Very high in vitamin C

# ADVENTUROUS JALAPENO

INGREDIENTS:
1 FRESH JALAPENO PEPPER
1 GREEN BELL PEPPER, DESEEDED
1 CUP ROMAINE LETTUCE
2 CUPS HONEYDEW MELON
1 CUP ICE
1 CUP WATER

170 CALORIES

Very low in saturated fat
No cholesterol
Low in sodium
High in dietary fiber
High in potassium
Very high in vitamin A
Very high in vitamin B6
Very high in vitamin C

# HELLO TANGELO

INGREDIENTS:
2 TANGELOS, PEELED
1 CUP ROMAINE LETTUCE
1 CUP GREEN GRAPES
2 KIWI FRUITS
1 CUP ICE
1 CUP WATER

300 CALORIES

Very low in saturated fat
No cholesterol
Very low in sodium
High in dietary fiber
High in potassium
Very high in vitamin B6
Very high in vitamin C

# FEELIN' DANDY

INGREDIENTS:
1 CUP DANDELION GREENS
1 CUP PINEAPPLE
1 APPLE
1 CUP ICE
1 CUP ORANGE JUICE

## 310 CALORIES

Very low in saturated fat
No cholesterol
Very low in sodium
High in dietary fiber
High in iron
Very high in manganese
Very high in vitamin A
Very high in vitamin B6
Very high in vitamin C

# BASIL BREEZE

INGREDIENTS:
1 CUP FRESH BABY SPINACH
1 SMALL BUNCH BASIL
1 CUP WATERMELON
1 CUP HONEYDEW MELON
1 CUP ICE
1 CUP UNSWEETENED ALMOND MILK

## 140 CALORIES

Very low in saturated fat
No cholesterol
Very high in calcium
High in manganese
High in magnesium
High in potassium
Very high in vitamin A
Very high in vitamin C
Very high in vitamin E

# GRAPE-ORANGE GALA

INGREDIENTS:
1 CUP GREEN GRAPES
1 CUP SWISS CHARD
2 APPLES
1 CUP ICE
1 CUP ORANGE JUICE

## 370 CALORIES

Very low in saturated fat
No cholesterol
Low in sodium
High in dietary fiber
High in vitamin A
Very high in vitamin B6
Very high in vitamin C

# NECTARINE NIRVANA

**INGREDIENTS:**
**3 NECTARINES, DESEEDED**
**1 CUP BABY SPINACH**
**1 CUP CANTALOUPE**
**1 CUP ICE**
**1 CUP WATER**

**250 CALORIES**

Very low in saturated fat
No cholesterol
Low in sodium
High in dietary fiber
High in niacin
High in potassium
Very high in vitamin A
Very high in vitamin C

# FLAXSEED FUSION

INGREDIENTS:
1 CUP ROMAINE LETTUCE
2 TABLESPOONS FLAXSEED
2 BANANAS
1 CUP GREEN GRAPES
1 GREEN APPLE
1 CUP ICE
1 CUP WATER

## 450 CALORIES

Low in saturated fat
No cholesterol
Very low in sodium
High in dietary fiber
High in manganese
Very high in vitamin B6
High in vitamin C

# MINT MANGO MAGIC

INGREDIENTS:
1 SMALL HANDFUL MINT
2 MANGOES, PEELED AND DESEEDED
1 CUP ROMAINE LETTUCE
1 CUP FRESH PINEAPPLE
1 CUP ICE
1 CUP COCONUT WATER

## 275 CALORIES

Very low in saturated fat
No cholesterol
Very high in manganese
High in vitamin A
High in vitamin B6
Very high in vitamin C

# BOK CHOY BERRY BLAST

INGREDIENTS:
1 ½ CUPS CHOPPED BOK CHOY
½ CUP STRAWBERRIES
½ CUP BLUEBERRIES
1 CUP FRESH PINEAPPLE
¼ CUP OATMEAL
1 CUP ICE
1 CUP WATER

240 CALORIES

Very low in saturated fat
No cholesterol
Low in sodium
High in dietary fiber
Very high in manganese
Very high in vitamin A
Very high in vitamin B6
Very high in vitamin C

# SPINACH SUNSET

INGREDIENTS:
2 APPLES
3 CELERY STALKS
1 CUP GREEN GRAPES
1 ½ CUPS BABY SPINACH
¼ CUP OATMEAL
1 CUP ICE
1 CUP WATER

## 350 CALORIES

Very low in saturated fat
No cholesterol
Low in sodium
High in dietary fiber
High in manganese
Very high in vitamin A
Very high in vitamin B6
Very high in vitamin C

# GOTTA SWEET DATE

## INGREDIENTS:
½ CUP DATES, HALVED AND PITTED
1 CUP ROMAINE LETTUCE
1 CUP ICE
1 CUP ALMOND MILK COCONUT MILK BLEND

## 300 CALORIES

Low in saturated fat
No cholesterol
Low in sodium
High in calcium
High in dietary fiber
High in vitamin B6
High in vitamin E

# GINGER BERRY BLASTER

INGREDIENTS:
1 CUP RASPBERRIES
1 CUP BLACKBERRIES
½ CUP STRAWBERRIES
1 TEASPOON FRESH GINGER
2 CUPS ROMAINE LETTUCE
1 CUP ICE
1 CUP WATER

## 270 CALORIES

Very low in saturated fat
No cholesterol
Very low in sodium
Very high in dietary fiber
High in iron
Very high in manganese
High in magnesium
High in potassium
Very high in vitamin B6
Very high in vitamin C

# BANANA BOAT

## INGREDIENTS:
2 FROZEN BANANAS
1 CUP PINEAPPLE
1 ½ CUPS KALE
1 CUP ICE
1 CUP UNSWEETENED COCONUT ALMOND MILK BLEND

## 390 CALORIES

Low in saturated fat
No cholesterol
Low in sodium
High in calcium
High in dietary fiber
Very high in manganese
High in potassium
Very high in vitamin A
Very high in vitamin B6
Very high in vitamin C
High in vitamin E

# CARROT MANGO CRUSH

INGREDIENTS:
3 CARROTS
2 MANGOES, PEELED AND DESEEDED
2 CUPS ROMAINE LETTUCE
1 CUP PINEAPPLE
1 CUP ICE
1 CUP WATER

310 CALORIES

Very low in saturated fat
No cholesterol
Low in sodium
High in dietary fiber
Very high in manganese
High in potassium
Very high in vitamin A
Very high in vitamin B6
Very high in vitamin C

# STRAWBERRY SWIRL

INGREDIENTS:
1 CUP STRAWBERRIES
½ CUP PINEAPPLE
1 RED DELICIOUS APPLE
1 CUP FRESH BABY SPINACH
1 CUP ICE
1 CUP WATER

190 CALORIES

Very low in saturated fat
No cholesterol
Low in sodium
High in dietary fiber
Very high in manganese
High in potassium
Very high in vitamin A
Very high in vitamin B6
Very high in vitamin C

# ALMOND APRICOT

INGREDIENTS:
5 MEDIUM APRICOTS, DESEEDED
½ CUP ALMONDS
1 TSP. ALMOND EXTRACT
1 CUP ROMAINE LETTUCE
1/2 CUP UNSWEETENED COCONUT ALMOND MILK
1 CUP ICE
1/2 CUP WATER

400 CALORIES

No cholesterol
Low in sodium
High in vitamin A
High in protein

# RICH RAPINI

INGREDIENTS:
1 AVOCADO, DESEEDED AND SCOOPED
1 CUP FRESH PINEAPPLE
1 ½ CUPS RAPINI
1 CUP ICE
1 CUP WATER

490 CALORIES

No cholesterol
Very low in sodium
High in dietary fiber
Very high in manganese
Very high in vitamin C

# IF YOU LIKE PINA COLADAS

INGREDIENTS:
1 CUP FRESH PINEAPPLE
¼ CUP UNSWEETENED COCONUT FLAKES [419845]
½ TSP. COCONUT EXTRACT
1 CUP ROMAINE LETTUCE
1 CUP ICE
1 CUP UNSWEETENED COCONUT ALMOND MILK

## 320 CALORIES

No cholesterol
Low in sodium
High in calcium
Very high in manganese
High in vitamin B6
Very high in vitamin C
High in vitamin E

# APRICOT ANTIOXIDANTS

INGREDIENTS:
3 APRICOTS, DESEEDED
½ CUP POMEGRANATE JUICE
1 LARGE APPLE
1 CUP RADISH GREENS
1 CUP ICE
1 CUP WATER

175 CALORIES

Very low in saturated fat
No cholesterol
Low in sodium
Very high in dietary fiber
High in potassium
Very high in vitamin A
Very high in vitamin B6
Very high in vitamin C

# BLACK CHERRY DETOX

INGREDIENTS:
1 CUP BLACK CHERRIES, PITTED
½ CUP STRAWBERRIES
2 CUPS DANDELION GREENS
1 CUP ICE
1 CUP WATER

190 CALORIES

Very low in saturated fat
No cholesterol
High in calcium
High in dietary fiber
High in iron
High in manganese
Very high in vitamin A
Very high in vitamin C

# SWEET CITRUS SUNRISE

INGREDIENTS:
1 TABLESPOON LEMON JUICE
2 ORANGES, PEELED AND SEGMENTED
½ CUP GRAPEFRUIT JUICE
1 CUP PINEAPPLE
2 CUPS RAPINI
1 CUP ICE
1 CUP WATER

## 345 CALORIES

Very low in saturated fat
No cholesterol
Low in sodium
High in dietary fiber
Very high in manganese
Very high in vitamin A
Very high in vitamin C

# REFRESHING CUCUMBER APPLE

INGREDIENTS:
2 LARGE CUCUMBERS
2 APPLES
½ CUP GREEN GRAPES
1 CUP ROMAINE LETTUCE
1 CUP ICE
1 CUP WATER

320 CALORIES

Very low in saturated fat
No cholesterol
Very low in sodium
High in dietary fiber
High in manganese
High in potassium
Very high in vitamin B6
Very high in vitamin C

# PRETTY POMEGRANATE

INGREDIENTS:
1 CUP PINEAPPLE
1 CUP POMEGRANATE JUICE
2 CUPS BABY SPINACH
1 CUP ICE
1 CUP WATER

240 CALORIES

Very low in saturated fat
No cholesterol
Low in sodium
Very high in manganese
High in potassium
Very high in vitamin A
Very high in vitamin C

# ORANGE DREAM

INGREDIENTS:
3 DATES, PITTED
2 ORANGES, PEELED AND SEGMENTED
2 CUPS ROMAINE LETTUCE
1 CUP ICE
1 CUP UNSWEETENED COCONUT ALMOND MILK

## 300 CALORIES

Low in saturated fat
No cholesterol
Low in sodium
Very high in calcium
High in dietary fiber
High in potassium
Very high in vitamin B6
Very high in vitamin C
High in vitamin E

# PLUM POWERHOUSE

INGREDIENTS:
4 PLUMS, PITTED
1 CUP PINEAPPLE
1 ½ CUPS RADISH GREENS
1 CUP ICE
1 CUP WATER

200 CALORIES

Very low in saturated fat
No cholesterol
Low in sodium
High in calcium
High in dietary fiber
Very high in manganese
High in potassium
Very high in vitamin A
Very high in vitamin C

# APPLE APRICOT CRUSH

INGREDIENTS:
5 APRICOTS, PITTED
2 APPLES
½ CUP FRESH PINEAPPLE
½ CUP GREEN GRAPES
1 CUP ROMAINE LETTUCE
1 CUP ICE
1 CUP WATER

350 CALORIES

Very low in saturated fat
No cholesterol
Very low in sodium
High in dietary fiber
Very high in manganese
High in vitamin A
Very high in vitamin B6
Very high in vitamin C

# STRAWBERRY VANILLA SOY

INGREDIENTS:
½ CUP STRAWBERRIES
½ CUP VANILLA SOYMILK
1 APPLE
2 BANANAS
1 CUP FRESH BABY SPINACH
1 CUP ICE
1 CUP WATER

## 385 CALORIES

Very low in saturated fat
No cholesterol
Low in sodium
High in dietary fiber
High in manganese
High in potassium
High in vitamin A
Very high in vitamin B6
Very high in vitamin C

# POMMELO PERFECTION

**INGREDIENTS:**
1 POMMELO, PEELED AND SEGMENTED
½ CUP GRAPEFRUIT JUICE
1 CUP PINEAPPLE
1 CUP MANDARIN ORANGE SLICES
1 CUP RAPINI
1 CUP ICE
1 CUP UNSWEETENED COCONUT ALMOND MILK

## 330 CALORIES

Low in saturated fat
No cholesterol
Low in sodium
High in calcium
Very high in manganese
Very high in vitamin A
Very high in vitamin B6
Very high in vitamin C
High in vitamin E

# SKINNY STRAWBERRY GUAVA

INGREDIENTS:
2 GUAVA FRUITS
½ CUP STRAWBERRIES
½ CUP PINEAPPLE
1 CUP DANDELION GREENS
1 CUP ICE
1 CUP WATER

150 CALORIES

Very low in saturated fat
No cholesterol
Low in sodium
Very high in dietary fiber
High in iron
Very high in manganese
Very high in vitamin A
Very high in vitamin C

# TANGY TANGERINE TWIST

INGREDIENTS:
3 TANGERINES, PEELED AND SEGMENTED
2 CUPS RAPINI
1 CUP ICE
1 CUP UNSWEETENED ALMOND MILK

350 CALORIES

Very low in saturated fat
No cholesterol
High in calcium
High in thiamin
Very high in vitamin A
Very high in vitamin C
High in vitamin E

# WATERMELON WORKOUT

INGREDIENTS:
1 CUP WATERMELON
½ CUP STRAWBERRIES
2 CELERY STALKS
1 ½ CUPS FRESH BABY SPINACH
½ CUP OATMEAL
1 CUP ICE
1 CUP UNSWEETENED ALMOND MILK

## 270 CALORIES

Low in saturated fat
No cholesterol
Very high in calcium
High in dietary fiber
Very high in manganese
High in magnesium
Very high in vitamin A
Very high in vitamin C
High in vitamin E

# ELDERBERRY ELIXIR

## INGREDIENTS:
1 CUP ELDERBERRIES
½ CUP BLUEBERRIES
¼ CUP POMEGRANATE JUICE
1 BANANA
2 CUPS ROMAINE LETTUCE
1 CUP ICE
1 CUP WATER

## 300 CALORIES

Very low in saturated fat
No cholesterol
Very low in sodium
Very high in dietary fiber
High in iron
High in potassium
Very high in vitamin B6
Very high in vitamin C

# RASPBERRY RHUBARB

## INGREDIENTS:
½ CUP RASPBERRIES
1 LARGE APPLE
½ CUP RHUBARB
1 CUP BABY SPINACH
1 CUP ICE
1 CUP WATER

## 170 CALORIES

Very low in saturated fat
No cholesterol
Low in sodium
Very high in dietary fiber
High in manganese
High in potassium
Very high in vitamin A
Very high in vitamin B6
Very high in vitamin C

# ORANG-O-TANGO

INGREDIENTS:
2 NAVEL ORANGES, PEELED AND SEGMENTED
1 BANANA
2 KIWI FRUITS
1 GREEN APPLE
2 CUPS ROMAINE LETTUCE
1 CUP ICE
1 CUP WATER

## 480 CALORIES

Very low in saturated fat
No cholesterol
Very low in sodium
High in dietary fiber
High in potassium
Very high in vitamin B6
Very high in vitamin C

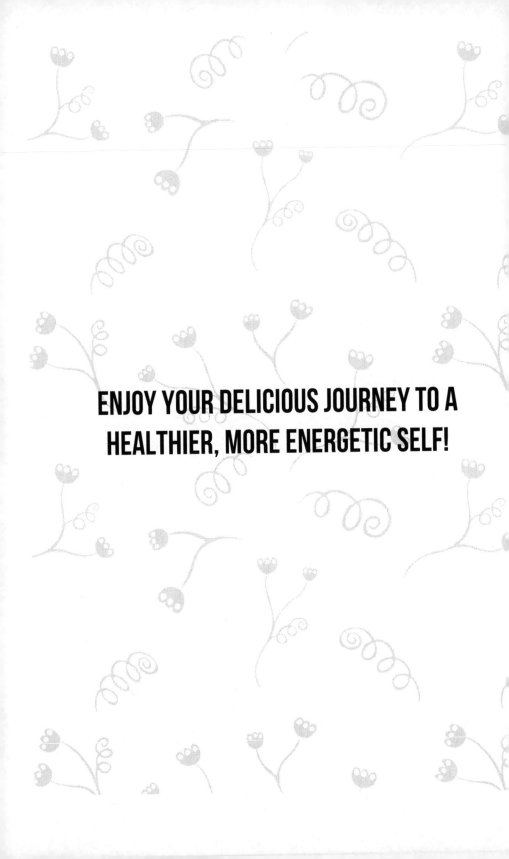

# ENJOY YOUR DELICIOUS JOURNEY TO A HEALTHIER, MORE ENERGETIC SELF!

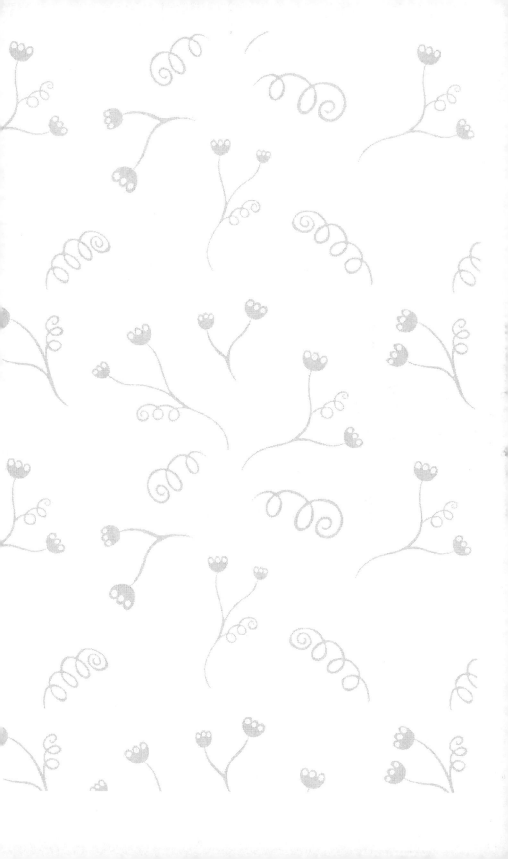

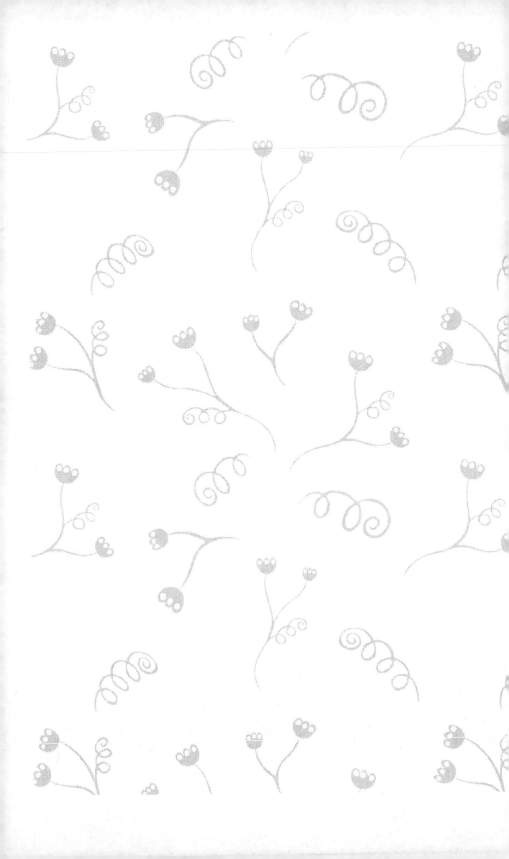

Made in the USA
Lexington, KY
19 March 2015